Index

Written By
James Wheeler
© 2018

<u>Introduction to the nut life</u>

Now this is the story of how my life got turned upside down, I'd like you to take a minute just sit right there I'll tell you how I….. Lost six and a half stone, 41 kg or 90 pounds in 3 months. I was 24 stone, I'm 6.4 and very broad so I hide it well but still very heavy!! Like most people, tried the gym but just felt a bit out of place and self-conscious which made it harder for me before I even got to the work out part, which was a struggle because I was so unfit and heavy that my body started to give up a couple of weeks in. Every time I tried I would pull a muscle or some other excuse would pop up and I would give myself a pass.

So now your like is this just another one of those stupid sob story things with a diet that was really the gym, that doesn't work or that demand that you don't eat anything with salt or something else that most people are just never going to be bothered to do because it's a massive pain in the

………………..

Anyhow this is not one of those, but it does require some commitment, this is a guide. I have written this to help you find your own balance, not only to lose the weight but keep it off for good.

The truth is that any diet is a challenge and the Squirrel Diet is no exception, on the bright side all you need to do is take it step by step and as I'm sure you have guessed start by replacing junk food and snacks with nuts and fruit, it's actually really easy, I'll show you in this guide and I promise not to write too much so that you don't make it to the end.

This is not a book or some epic story to read, with all the facts about nuts and their benefits and all the jargon the good the bad…..boring….. I could have made this 50 plus pages but be honest would you have read it?.......Yer that's what I thought, not least of which I'm not a nutritionist, just a guy that had an idea for his own diet, having tried a number of others and failed miserably at them, now I'm trying to help other people like me.

If you're allergic to nuts why are you reading this? Also if you have any pre-existing medical conditions ask a doctor before you start. (see page 50 for full disclaimer) Now the disclaimers are over. This is meant to be fun and the best way for this to work is if you to take in the information, so this guide will need to be interesting and funny….. so….sorry about that…

This is about small steps, little changes that will add up to a big difference, in this guide we will go through these steps from changes to breakfast to changes to drunk you eating peanuts over a kebab or my go to 4 rounds of toast and cheesy beans!!

General guidelines to a good nut

So….don't just eat a load of salted peanuts instead of a packet of crisps, what's the point, I can tell you now that you will be hungry….you are on a diet and the first two weeks of each stage are the worst.

The First guideline is to have a handful of relatively healthy nuts when you're hungry, i.e. cashew nuts they were my choice but get a variety and find the ones that you like or just get a mixed bag that's the easy way, they will need to be just nuts not salted or roasted just plain old boring nuts! Some of the supermarkets do mixed bags of fruit and nuts that are a good call.

Two, get some fruit that you like, bananas are good and grapes work a treat to help curb your hunger, this is the theme for the whole diet, it is about curbing your hunger not stuffing your face with fruit and nuts…. It is about taking the edge off and slowly making changes to the way you eat and what you eat without overly concerning yourself with calorie counting, in my experience calorie counting is a hiding to nothing, ultimately if you eat a chocolate bar and then count the calories you still ate a chocolate bar, you are supposed to be on a diet, can somebody please explain that to me, it is not how many calories you have, but how to avoid having the calories in the first place.

Three, don't worry about the scales!! They don't come into play for the first couple of weeks, this is not a diet that will have an immediate impact, though if you go straight to Stage Three you will lose a lot of weight very quickly, it is not something you should do lightly it is hard and without the build-up through this guide you might not do it for long.

That is what happened to me, I discovered that it is better to change things slowly and let myself adjust to the new dynamic before taking the next step, you should only start keeping track of your weight after you start to feel thinner. Your clothes will start to fit better, then get on the scales and you will probably fall off them in shock, for me that was about five weeks in, after I had started Stage Two but we will get to that.

Four, this diet is not quick and easy it is an endurance test and if you are like me, you will probably always be on some form of it for the rest of your life. The beauty of this is that you find what works for you and you add it to your life. Mine was breakfast, I went from being a cereal and toast person to having a banana and some nuts for breakfast. You will be shocked how far you get by just changing that one thing.

Five, don't worry about religiously sticking to your diet as there will be days when you're just going to be like "screw this". The trick is not to let that become a pattern, let that one day or one meal get you through the next week, it's about using that feeling of guilt to your advantage, giving yourself a reason to not break your diet. An example is that today I was up really early to catch a train, I was driving past McDonald's and thought to myself I want a McDonald's breakfast so I had one, but now I won't have anything like that again for at least two weeks because I can guilt myself with that one meal.

After a while when you have settled into the diet around week six you will need to start finding a balance. If you have a meal that is not so good for you or you have a fat day, at some point in the next three or four days you will have to pay for that, this diet is about patience and being consistent so if you have a burger one day you have a minimal lunch the next so on so forth.

Six, NO SNACKS!!! Unless its nuts, even then only a handful, if you have small hands that's your problem.

Seven, hunger is your friend, I know it's uncomfortable and I know it's not a pleasant feeling but if you're hungry your body will use your fat stores and if like me, you're not a fan of working out and going to the gym everyday, then you will just have to learn to embrace your hunger.

Eight, drinking water is good for you it will help push your hunger down and water is the only thing other than coffee and tea that you should drink. (Because mornings are the worst, no sugar though that's cheating!) That means, no fizzy drinks (fizzy water is a good replacement) and no concentrate either, one of the best ways I found to get round this is to mix fresh orange juice with fizzy water, so if you have to have some taste or you just need something other than plain water there is a good little trick to get you through that craving.

Nine, competition is good! None of this new age everyone wins rubbish, back to the 80's, winning is the only thing and everyone else can suck it!!! Get some of your friends together or use Instagram and Facebook, I have set up a Facebook page and Instagram account, and I will try to use them but I am not the best with all this social media stuff and I've got a job so bear with me. You don't need me to have a competition to see who can lose the most weight in 3 or 4 months. The pages will be there so you can communicate with each other as well as me, but the best way is going to be if you get your friends involved and try and have some fun with it.

The reason for the competition is very simple, it will help keep you on track and you can help each other through some of the more difficult parts of the diet, plus it can be fun. A little bit of banter goes a long way for lifting your mood which then makes everything easier or at least that's what I found.

Ten, you want to take your time to lose weight you can't expect results in the first day or even the first week, it will take time but have some faith, stick to it and you will see the results! This is not a diet that will give you an arbitrary time scale and set goals that you have to achieve, take it at your own pace, don't be pressured and bullied this is a guide not a plan. It is for you to develop your own plan. I am not here to spoon feed you I'm here to "show you the door, you have to be the one to walk through it" Yes I did just quote the Matrix.

One last thing that needs to be addressed before we start, cravings are the worst thing for a diet!! They will win sooner or later so last as long as you can. There are two ways that I found help deal with cravings, all you need to do is find a healthier option and before you say that won't work have you ever actually looked? Take nuts, for instance, you will find that for the most part you're craving is actually hunger.

The best way I found to deal with them was to find a way to hold your cravings at bay, mine was a chocolate biscuit with a cup of tea at the end of the day, I know how very English of me, focusing on that end of day treat helped me work through a lot of the cravings that I ran into and could help you in your day to day life, find your treat and use it.

There are also some healthier options that tasted nice if you're missing the chocolate bars. There are loads of different healthy eating products you just have to look for them, find the one that you like best and use it to help you push the craving aside; this does not mean eat three in a row it means eat one a day maximum!!

<u>*Drunken Squirrels*</u>

<u>*(If your under 18 don't read this you shouldn't be drinking anyway ;)*</u>

Ok so drunk you doesn't give a **** that you're on a diet, drunk you is only after one thing….FOOD!! Which normally ends up being something very very bad for you, of course you shouldn't be drinking because you're on a diet, which we all know won't stop us and it shouldn't, sometimes you just need to go out with some mates and have a few beers. I would say that this should not be a regular occurrence especially in the first four or five weeks the diet.

On the whole, it's no good for you, and you should try to moderate how much your drinking just as a general life rule because drinking is "bad for you" but also a lot of fun especially on a night out!

So now comes the advice, do not buy any fast food!! A couple of hours before you go out, go to your local supermarket or shop and get yourself some roasted and salted peanuts, mix them together and wait until you get home, then drunk you can stuff his/her face with as many peanuts as you can possibly handle. An added bonus is that these might help lessen your hangover!

The next day just give yourself a pass, because being on a diet on a hangover day is never going to work so consider this your out of jail free card, whatever you want, whatever you need, get yourself back to some sort of normality. Just pick up from where we left off the next day.

After all, what's the point in losing all that weight feeling more confident, being happier in yourself and then not going out and enjoying it? Trust me that is what will happen if you managed to stick to this diet, it will take time but in the end, the results will speak for themselves.

<u>To Start</u>

Right so the way that this works, I have broken the diet into three stages, each stage has a breakfast, lunch and dinner. A stage has no set timescale; there are no hard and fast rules, this is the path that you have to decide for yourself, if you're happy with just doing stage 1 and you are feeling the results that you want by all means stick to it.

Each stage will get progressively... well worse, or better depending on your point of view. There are a couple of things to go over. For me, each stage lasted for about a month, so I would say four to six weeks is a good call, any more than that and I feel like you will just be stagnating, any less than that I don't think that you've managed to adjust. The idea of each stage is to shock your body into using your fat stores while lowering your calorie intake and still providing nutrition.

Set a goal, this is important you will need a target to shoot for, but make sure it is on your terms, once you have hit it take a break, evaluate how you feel not what you think other people think. This is ultimately about you, where you are happy? When do you feel you are comfortable? This will not get you abs and that perfect beach body, what it will do is give you the confidence to hit the gym and show you that it is not hard to lose weight, it is not an insurmountable challenge, and that cycle of feeling unhappy with your body and eating your feelings is so easy to break.

Last of all I know I said there is no exercise needed and there isn't "everything before the word BUT is horse ****" doing some exercise will go a long way to helping you achieve your goal and I'm not talking going to the gym everyday more like take a walk in the park once a week, get your body moving start using it, stop sitting on your ass!! If you do decide to hit the gym it should help a lot, I didn't, as of me writing this I am about to restart and I will be doing exercise in conjunction with the diet but I am going to try and do this on social media, just not sure how, probably Facebook, search for the Squirrel Diet and it will be there.

<u>*Stage One*</u>

Breakfast

Breakfast is the most important meal of the day, especially in this diet. As it is the first thing that you will change and ultimately will stay the same throughout all the stages of this diet.

All you need to do is have a piece of fruit and some nuts, that's it nothing special, find a fruit that you like, I generally have a banana but it is nice to mix it up especially after a while, oranges, apples I even found avocados to be quite a nice one, like I said this isn't really difficult to achieve and it sounds very simple, that's because it is very simple.

Now if you're like "I don't have much for breakfast anyway" then that's fine but still switch what you are having which, I imagine is some sort of yoghurt and just have a piece of fruit and handful of nuts.

The issues that most people including myself run into is that you will snack in between meals, this is something that you just need to keep track of and stop yourself from doing. That chocolate biscuit with your cup of tea in the office or if there's some cake going around or that pack of crisps that you demolish on your break time. If you do get really hungry then just have another handful of nuts or a piece of fruit, No more snacks!

Lunch

So lunch….well this is a bit more challenging especially if you are busy, look there is nothing wrong with a sandwich, it's the packet of crisps and the fizzy drink that are the problem.

Try changing those two things instead of the crisps get some houmous and carrots or a little bag of fruit, don't get me wrong in this stage your lunch can stay relatively the same. At the moment it's just about starting to be more conscious of what you eat, then trying to make some small changes in the first weeks of the diet, don't worry about lunch it's the breakfast that you need to concentrate on.

After you've managed to get used to the breakfast then you really do need to start thinking about scaling back some aspects of your lunch, if you just want to go for it and honestly that's what I did, cut out the drinks and crisps altogether. I've already mentioned houmous and carrots which are actually quite a good filler and some fruit, when you do get a hankering get some crisps indulge yourself once or twice a week.

Again if you don't eat much lunch then try cutting out the sweets and sugary drinks, no snaking when the hunger gets too much, push through it have a glass of water when it gets really bad have another handful of nuts!

Dinner

In stage one have a normal dinner, whatever it would generally be, maybe try and cut out the takeaways and fast food and again start thinking to yourself "how can I make this healthier" but there is no rush. The reason dinner doesn't change is that it will help you cope with the rest of the challenges in the diet. If you are ever struggling and you will at some point just think about dinner, use that to push through "I only have to make it another couple of hours" it's an effective motivation to help you out.

<u>Stage Two</u>

Breakfast- See Stage One

Lunch

This is where things start getting a bit more difficult, there are no sandwiches it will be mostly soups, salads and lean meats. Think about the healthy food that you like…….. Or can stand to eat and obviously with some nuts thrown in.

There are no crisps, chocolate bars or fizzy drinks! If you do have a bit of a sweet tooth, try raisins or even better get a mixed bag of nuts and raisins, but for the most part, you are just going to have to deal with it.

For me, lunch was always a challenge, so I tended to do more grazing with the mainstay of my lunch being roasted meat generally chicken. What I tended to do after the first week or so was make my lunch the night before rather than buy it, because I had a bit more control over how much food I had and it was also cheaper. On a side note I did find that sometimes I just needed a piece of crusty bread to help pull my meal together and again rather than getting the whole sandwich with the mayonnaise or butter I used olive oil and had a deconstructed sandwich. This is where it all comes down to personal preference, you need to go and find the food that you like that is healthier and find ways to make what you do like healthier.

You will find at this stage that you will be hungry more often, this is where those packs of nuts I keep banging on about really come into play, because you will go through one of them a day. The ones that I got were 170g of fruit and nuts (super nutty with raisins), without them I wouldn't have lasted a week and you will find out during this stage why it is called the Squirrel Diet, but I do have to remind you not to go overboard. Do not stuff your face with nuts, it is about curbing the hunger. This is why I got the 170g packs because it already put a limit on the amount that I can have, it is also a good little trick to make sure that you don't go over the top.

Dinner

This is where things start to get really boring; I am warning you now that the food groups you can eat are:

Chicken

Fish

Rice

Vegetables

Yeah that's it…….. I know there is not a whole lot there but then it is a diet. The idea is to have one piece of chicken breast or plain fish not breaded or battered. I know what you were thinking!! (If you are craving a steak try a tuna steak not the same but very nice) with half a bag of mixed vegetables and some rice. Again I got the microwaveable packs of rice as they are a set amount and there are loads of different types which could add a new dimension to a very bland meal plan.

I know it's boring but the thing is boring works, boring will get you to that goal weight and make you appreciate the nice foods in your life so much more. There are some good ways to switch it up. Stir-fry with vegetables and prawns with a bit of sweet chilli sauce. I make a mean sweet chilli king prawn stir-fry. Have a look on the internet find some Youtubers that you like and try their ideas. The above is just what I did and so long as the food is healthy you are on the right track!

There are also loads of healthy ready meals that you can have; I tried only to have them every couple of days just to mix up my meals as they do get repetitive.

Stage three

Breakfast- See Stage One

Lunch

Well, you know that bag of 170g nuts I told you about…..yer that's now your lunch. No, I am not taking the **** that's it, well you can add some fruit like an apple or orange, if you are struggling get a little pack of hummus and carrots, I found that helped me. Hey, no pain no gain.

If you do have to revert back to stage two lunch for a bit that's fine, I did try to alternate between the two stages, that is the best way that I found because the stage three lunch is hard, only a bag of nuts and some fruit for the day is not fun, but this is where you will start seeing major results. Remember to have water it will help.

Dinner

How can dinner get any worse….well take out the rice and add some vegetables that's it. It is not hard…….I'm lying, it is just wait for it, you will hate me for this but by the end I'll get a thank you.

Just as a warning stage three is not for the faint-hearted, this is for the people who are struggling to reach their goal weight or have a lot more weight to lose. If you only wanted to lose two stone by now you should have done it. Stage two is more than enough to get you to that goal.

Stage three is for the people who have set a four or five stone goal, how healthy it is in the long run, is very much up for debate, but if you do have a lot of weight to lose this is realistically the only way to do it, without massive amounts of exercise. The irony being that you're probably too unfit to actually do any real useful exercise, this is where I was as I said I was so unfit that I would just hurt myself in the gym.

This stage requires a lot of willpower, the other two stages have been about mentally preparing you to be able to deal with the hunger that you're going to face and developing better overall eating habits. The nuts help and when I was doing this stage I did tend to have two of those bags of the 170 grams a day but trust me when I tell you it is a challenge.

After a couple of weeks I personally started to struggle in this stage, it is a lot….. well actually it's not enough…. but you know what I mean, I tended to switch between stage two and three from week to week, trying to compartmentalise the stage as getting through a week is easier than a month.

At this point if you have stuck to the diet you would have seen huge changes, now comes the hard part, how do you keep the weight off because losing the weight sadly is not the greatest challenge. Keeping it off it's a lifelong fight. This diet will have shown you how easy it is to lose the weight.

It's ok to put on half a stone over the winter and then in February just do stage one and two to lose it. The truth is the weight is even easier to put back on than it is to lose, what you need to do is figure out what out of all three of these stages fits into your life the best and change it. I would suggest breakfast that's what I did. It has helped me control my weight and myself. Along with the eating habits that I developed and that you will develop during this diet, all of this will help you maintain your goal weight and the confidence you gain from it.

Like I said short and sweet, not a book, a guide. Now it's up to you! I have done my bit, have fun with it and share your results with me and everyone else!!! #bustanut#settinggoals

Squirrels on Paper

So apparently to do a paperback version of the Squirrel Diet it needs to be at least 24 pages long, (only just realised that I can set the size of the book to A5😱) which is pretty much the opposite of the point of the diet. It's meant to be short, easy to read, easy to understand and easy to follow, not over extended, repetitive and boring.

So rather than 10 pages of squirrel pictures which was genuinely my first thought, I've decided to make the next few pages a bit more useful to you, to start with, it will be a diary.

I know, before you start, "I'm not keeping a diary" I don't mean a day by day long drawn out essay, everyday that you're doing the diet, I mean a once a week, sit down on the Sunday for 10 minutes, write down your successes and your failures and the things you struggled with that week, this will help you keep track of what you're doing and areas that you can improve. Ultimately, as with anything in life that is about commitment, losing weight is a challenge there are no pills to take no shortcuts. The more time you invest in this diet the more likely you are to see it through and make the changes that you want or need to make to your life.

As with everything in the squirrel diet it's totally up to you, use this don't use this, if you don't think it's going to help you then don't do it, having had some time to think about it, this is what I did although it wasn't really a diary. I did make notes not necessarily on how I'd been doing but more on what I'd been eating and how much, different ready meals that I liked, healthy eating bars that helps curb my cravings, as everyone is different in this world, some of the things that I did won't help other people and some of them will.

This diary might help you find your own balance. The next bit of the paperback where there's a section for you to develop your own guidelines that are specific to you not generalise rules to follow, but an individualised plan that will not only help you lose weight but maintain your goal weight for the rest of your life.

As I said before, I chose to change my breakfast and that is my own personal guideline I have fruit for breakfast small healthy-ish lunch whatever I want for dinner and I haven't put any weight on for 6 months.

I know I said I was going to restart my diet when I launch the Kindle version, but life had other plans and it is still my intention to do that and I will be doing it on Facebook and Instagram and putting out videos and developing content, but as of right now I'm not sure when that will be, hopefully around October time, but until then I think I'm going to be too busy, hence why it's taking me so long to actually sit down at the weekend and write the rest of this out.

You're weight………………..

You're Goal…………………

Squirrel Diary

<u>*Stage 1*</u>

Week 1

Week 2

Week 3

Week 4

<u>*Stage 2*</u>

Week 1

Week 2

You're weight…………..

Week 3

Week 4

You're weight…………

Stage 3

Week 1

Week 2

You're weight............

Week 3

Week 4

Did you make it? …………………..

What is your weight now? …………………

You're Guidelines

Use what you have learnt from all the above to develop you own plan that fits your needs and use the things you found out about yourself through doing this diet to develop your own guidelines that will give you the body you want for the rest of your life!

1. ___________________________________

____

____

____

____

____

____

____

2.

3.

4.

5.

6.

7.

8.

9.

10.

Me Before and After in the Same Suite, Shirt &Shoes

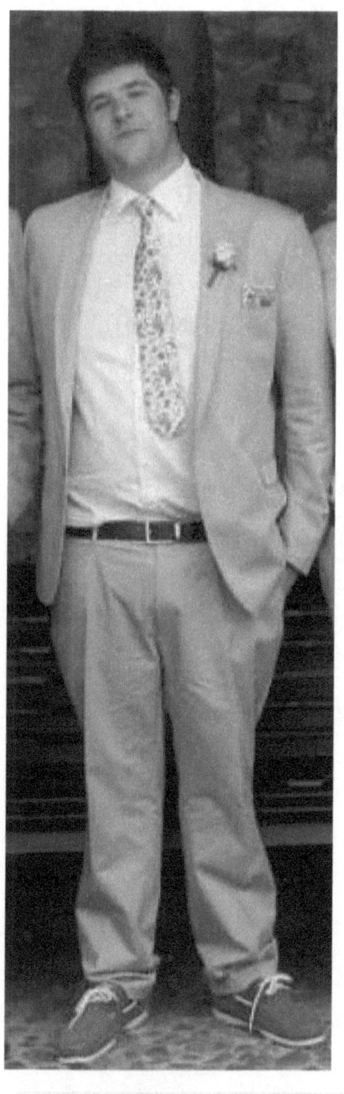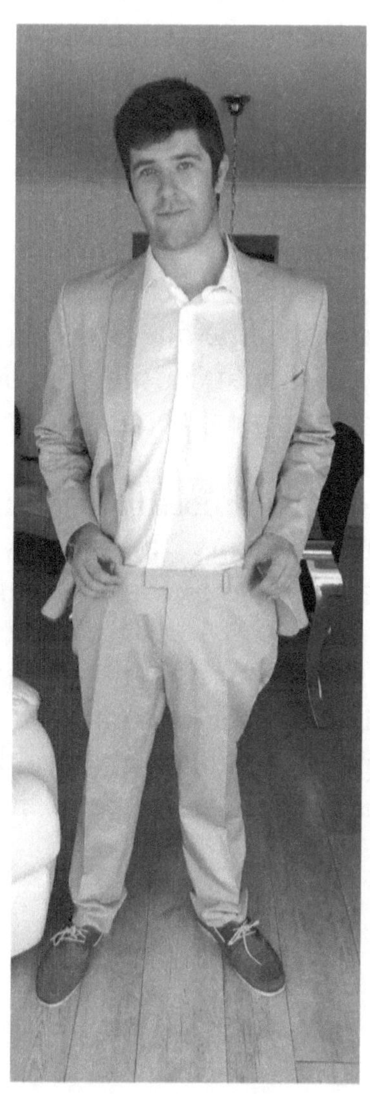

Disclaimer

I hate that I have to do this disclaimer stuff but some people will always try it on.

Before starting any diet, you should speak to your doctor. You must not rely on the information in this book as an alternative to medical advice from your doctor or other professional healthcare providers. If you have any specific questions about any medical matter you should consult your doctor or other professional healthcare providers.

This book does not guarantee results and is not a tested theory, this is just what happened for the author and how it was achieved.

The author does not accept any responsibility or liability for any other person or person's physical and mental health and well-being arising from the use of the diet.